MedicalCenter.com

The Key Facts on Alzheimer's Disease

Everything You Need to Know About Alzheimer's Disease

-Usable Medical Information for the Patient-

By Patrick W. Nee

www.MedicalCenter.com

Published by:

MedicalCenter.com

96 Walter Street/ Suite 200

Boston, MA 02131, USA

Tel: 617-354-7722

www.MedicalCenter.com

manager@medicalcenter.com

Copyright © 2013 by PWN

"Key Facts" is a TradeMark.

All Rights are reserved under International, Pan-American, and Pan-Asian Conventions. No part of this book may be reproduced in any form without the written permission of the publisher. All rights vigorously enforced.

Table of Contents

Chapter 1: What Is Alzheimer's Disease?

Chapter 2: Causes and Risk Factors

Chapter 3: Symptoms and Diagnosis

Chapter 4: Prevention

Chapter 5: Treatments

Chapter 6: Research

Chapter 7: Participating in Research

Chapter 8: Additional Resources

Chapter 9: Frequently Asked Questions

Chapter 1: What Is Alzheimer's Disease?

Alzheimer's disease is a brain disease that slowly destroys memory and thinking skills and, eventually, the ability to carry out the simplest tasks. It begins slowly and gets worse over time. Currently, it has no cure.

A Common Cause of Dementia

Alzheimer's disease is the most common cause of dementia among older people. Dementia is a loss of thinking, remembering, and reasoning skills that interferes with a person's daily life and activities. Dementia ranges in severity from the mild stage, when it is just beginning to affect a person's functioning, to the severe stage, when the person must depend completely on others for basic care.

Estimates vary, but experts suggest that as many as 5.1 million people in the United States may have Alzheimer's disease. Symptoms usually begin after age 60, and the risk of developing the disease increases with age. While younger people -- in their 30s, 40s, and 50s -- may get Alzheimer's disease, it is much less common. It is important to note that Alzheimer's disease is not a normal part of aging.

The course of Alzheimer's disease—which symptoms appear and how quickly changes occur—varies from person to person. The time from diagnosis to death varies, too. It can be as little as 3 or 4 years if the person is over 80 years old when diagnosed or as long as 10 years or more if the person is younger.

Memory Problems

Memory problems are typically one of the first signs of Alzheimer's disease. People with Alzheimer's have trouble doing everyday things like driving a car, cooking a meal, or paying bills. They may ask the same questions over and over, get lost easily, lose things or put them in odd places, and find even simple things confusing. Some people become worried, angry, or violent.

Not all people with memory problems have Alzheimer's disease. Mild forgetfulness can be a normal part of aging. Some people may notice that it takes longer to learn new things, remember certain words, or find their glasses.

Sometimes memory problems are related to health issues that are treatable. For example, medication side effects, vitamin B12 deficiency, or liver or kidney disorders can lead to memory loss or possibly dementia. Emotional problems, such as stress, anxiety, or depression, can also make a person more forgetful and may be mistaken for dementia.

Mild Cognitive Impairment

Some older people with memory or other thinking problems have a condition called mild cognitive impairment, or MCI. MCI can be an early sign of Alzheimer's, but not everyone with MCI will develop Alzheimer's disease. People with MCI can still take care of themselves and do their normal activities.

Signs of MCI may include

- losing things often
- forgetting to go to events and appointments
- having more trouble coming up with words than other people the same age.

If you or someone in your family thinks your forgetfulness is getting in the way of your normal routine, it's time to see your doctor. Seeing the doctor when you first start having memory problems can help you find out what's causing your forgetfulness.

What Happens to the Brain in Alzheimer's?

Alzheimer's disease is named after Dr. Alois Alzheimer, a German doctor. In 1906, Dr. Alzheimer noticed changes in the brain tissue of a woman who had died of an unusual mental illness. He found many abnormal clumps (now called amyloid plaques) and tangled bundles of fibers (now called neurofibrillary tangles). Plaques and tangles in the brain are two of the main features of Alzheimer's disease. The third is loss of connections between nerve cells in the brain.

Although we still don't know how Alzheimer's disease begins, it seems likely that damage to the brain starts 10 years or more before problems become obvious. During the earliest stage of Alzheimer's, people are free of symptoms, but harmful changes are taking place in the brain. Abnormal protein deposits form plaques and tangles in the brain. Once-healthy nerve cells lose their ability to function and communicate with each other, and eventually they die.

As nerve cells in the brain die, parts of the brain begin to shrink. By the final stage of Alzheimer's, damage is widespread, and brain tissue has shrunk significantly.

Chapter 2: Causes and Risk Factors

Causes Not Fully Understood

Scientists do not yet fully understand what causes Alzheimer's disease. It is likely that the causes include some mix of genetic, environmental, and lifestyle factors. These factors affect each person differently.

Research shows that Alzheimer's disease causes changes in the brain years and even decades before the first symptoms appear, so even people who seem free of the disease today may be at risk. Scientists are developing sophisticated tests to help identify who is most likely to develop symptoms of Alzheimer's. Ultimately, they hope to prevent or delay dementia in these high-risk individuals.

Risk Factors

Some risk factors for Alzheimer's, like age and genetics, cannot be controlled. Other factors that may play a role in the development of the disease—such as how much a person exercises or socializes—can be changed.

Lifestyle factors, such as diet and physical exercise, and long-term health conditions, like high blood pressure and diabetes, might also play a role in the risk of developing

Alzheimer's disease. For more information, see the chapter entitled "Prevention."

Older Age—The Biggest Risk Factor

Increasing age is the most important known risk factor for Alzheimer's disease. The number of people with the disease doubles every 5 years beyond age 65. Nearly half of people age 85 and older may have Alzheimer's. These facts are significant because the number of older adults is growing.

Genetics

There are two types of Alzheimer's disease—early-onset and late-onset.

- Early-onset Alzheimer's is a rare form of the disease that occurs in people age 30 to 60. Most of these cases are early-onset familial Alzheimer's disease, an inherited disease caused by mutations, or changes, in certain genes.
- Most people with Alzheimer's disease have late-onset Alzheimer's, which usually develops after age 60. No obvious family pattern is seen in most of these cases, but

genetic factors appear to increase a person's risk.

Many studies have linked the apolipoprotein E gene to late-onset Alzheimer's. One form of this gene, APOE ε4, increases a person's risk of getting the disease. But many people who get Alzheimer's do not have the APOE ε4 gene, and some people with the gene never get Alzheimer's.

Scientists have identified a number of other genes in addition to APOE ε4 that may increase a person's risk for late-onset Alzheimer's. Knowing about these genes can help researchers more effectively test possible treatments and prevention strategies in people who are at risk of developing Alzheimer's -- ideally, before symptoms appear.

Chapter 3: Symptoms and Diagnosis

Alzheimer's disease varies from person to person so not everyone will have the same symptoms. Also, the disease progresses faster in some people than in others. In general, though, Alzheimer's takes many years to develop and becomes increasingly severe over time.

Memory Problems -- A Common Early Sign

Memory problems are typically one of the first signs of Alzheimer's disease. However, not all memory problems are caused by Alzheimer's. If you or someone in your family thinks your forgetfulness is getting in the way of your normal routine, it's time to see your doctor. He or she can find out what's causing these problems.

A person in the early (mild) stage of Alzheimer's disease may

- find it hard to remember things
- ask the same questions over and over
- get lost
- lose things or put them in odd places
- have trouble handling money and paying bills

- take longer than normal to finish daily tasks
- have some mood and personality changes.

Other thinking problems besides memory loss may be the first sign of Alzheimer's disease. A person may have

- trouble finding the right words
- vision and spatial issues
- impaired reasoning or judgment.

Later Signs of Alzheimer's

As Alzheimer's disease progresses to the moderate stage, memory loss and confusion grow worse, and people may have problems recognizing family and friends. Other symptoms at this stage may include

- difficulty learning new things and coping with new situations
- trouble carrying out tasks that involve multiple steps, like getting dressed
- impulsive behavior
- forgetting the names of common things
- hallucinations, delusions, or paranoia
- wandering away from home.

Symptoms of Severe Alzheimer's

As Alzheimer's disease becomes more severe, people lose the ability to communicate. They may sleep more, lose weight, and have trouble swallowing. Often they are incontinent—they cannot control their bladder and/or bowels. Eventually, they need total care.

Benefits of Early Diagnosis

An early, accurate diagnosis of Alzheimer's disease helps people and their families plan for the future. It gives them time to discuss care options, find support, and make legal and financial arrangements while the person with Alzheimer's can still take part in making decisions. Also, even though no medicine or other treatment can stop or slow the disease, early diagnosis offers the best chance to treat the symptoms.

How Alzheimer's Is Diagnosed

The only definitive way to diagnose Alzheimer's disease is to find out whether plaques and tangles exist in brain tissue. To look at brain tissue, doctors perform a brain autopsy, an examination of the brain done after a person dies.

Doctors can only make a diagnosis of "possible" or "probable" Alzheimer's disease while a person is alive.

Doctors with special training can diagnose Alzheimer's disease correctly up to 90 percent of the time. Doctors who can diagnose Alzheimer's include geriatricians, geriatric psychiatrists, and neurologists. A geriatrician specializes in the treatment of older adults. A geriatric psychiatrist specializes in mental problems in older adults. A neurologist specializes in brain and nervous system disorders.

To diagnose Alzheimer's disease, doctors may

- ask questions about overall health, past medical problems, ability to carry out daily activities, and changes in behavior and personality
- conduct tests to measure memory, problem solving, attention, counting, and language skills
- carry out standard medical tests, such as blood and urine tests
- perform brain scans to look for anything in the brain that does not look normal.

Test results can help doctors know if there are other possible causes of the person's symptoms. For example, thyroid problems, drug reactions, depression, brain tumors, head injury, and blood-vessel disease in the brain can cause symptoms similar to those of Alzheimer's. Many of these other conditions can be treated successfully.

New Diagnostic Methods Being Studied

Researchers are exploring new ways to help doctors diagnose Alzheimer's disease earlier and more accurately. Some studies focus on changes in a person's memory, language, and other mental functions. Others look at changes in blood, spinal fluid, and brain-scan results that may detect Alzheimer's years before symptoms appear.

Chapter 4: Prevention

Currently, no medicines or other treatments are known to prevent Alzheimer's disease, but scientists are studying many possibilities. These possibilities include lifestyle factors such as exercise and physical activity, a healthy diet, and mentally stimulating activities.

In addition to lifestyle factors, scientists have found clues that some long-term health conditions, like heart disease, high blood pressure, and diabetes, are related to Alzheimer's disease. It's possible that controlling these conditions will reduce the risk of developing Alzheimer's.

Exercise and Physcial Activity

Studies show that exercise and other types of physical activity are good for our hearts, waistlines, and ability to carry out everyday activities. Research suggests that exercise may also play a role in reducing risk for Alzheimer's disease.

Animal studies show that exercise increases both the number of small blood vessels that supply blood to the brain and the number of connections between nerve cells in older rats and mice. In addition, researchers have found that exercise raises the level of a nerve growth factor (a protein key to brain health) in an area of the brain that is important to memory and learning. Researchers have also shown that exercise can stimulate the human brain's ability to maintain old network connections and make new ones.

Diet and Dietary Supplements

A number of studies suggest that eating certain foods may help keep the brain healthy—and that others can be harmful. A diet that includes lots of fruits, vegetables, and whole grains and is low in fat and added sugar can reduce the risk of heart disease and diabetes. Researchers are looking at whether a healthy diet also can help prevent Alzheimer's.

One study reported that people who ate a "Mediterranean diet" had a 28 percent lower risk of developing MCI (mild cognitive impairment) and a 48 percent lower risk of progressing from MCI to Alzheimer's disease. (MCI often, but not always, leads to Alzheimer's dementia.) A Mediterranean diet includes vegetables, legumes, fruits, cereals, fish, olive oil, and low amounts of saturated fats, dairy products, meat, and poultry.

Other research has looked at the effect on brain health of several different vitamins and dietary supplements. One area of research focuses on antioxidants, natural substances that appear to fight damage caused by molecules called free radicals. Other studies are looking at a compound called resveratrol, which is found in red grapes and red wine. A clinical trial supported by the National Institute on Aging is testing resveratrol in people with Alzheimer's disease.

Chronic Diseases

Age-related diseases and conditions—such as vascular disease, high blood pressure, heart disease, and diabetes—may increase the risk of Alzheimer's. Many studies are looking at whether this risk can be reduced by preventing or controlling these diseases and conditions.

For example, one clinical trial is looking at how lowering blood pressure to or below current recommended levels may affect cognitive decline and the development of MCI and Alzheimer's disease. Participants are older adults with high systolic (upper number) blood pressure who have a history of heart disease or stroke, or are at risk for those conditions.

Diabetes is another disease that has been linked to Alzheimer's. Past research suggests that abnormal insulin production contributes to Alzheimer's-related brain changes. (Insulin is the hormone involved in diabetes.) Diabetes treatments have been tested in people with Alzheimer's, but the results have not been conclusive.

Keeping the Brain Active

Keeping the mind sharp—through social engagement or intellectual stimulation—is associated with a lower risk of Alzheimer's disease. Activities like working, volunteering, reading, going to lectures, and playing computer and other games are being studied to see if they might help prevent Alzheimer's.

One clinical trial is testing the impact of formal cognitive training, with and without physical exercise, in people with MCI to see if it can prevent or delay Alzheimer's disease. Other trials are underway in healthy older adults to see if exercise and/or cognitive training (for example, a demanding video game) can delay or prevent age-related cognitive decline.

Chapter 5: Treatments

Medications Can Treat Symptoms

There is no known cure for Alzheimer's disease, but there are medicines that can treat symptoms of the disease. Most Alzheimer's medicines work best for people in the mild or moderate stages of the disease. For example, they can keep memory loss from getting worse for a time. Other medicines may help behavioral symptoms, such as trouble sleeping or feeling worried or depressed. All of these medicines may have side effects and may not work for everyone.

A person with Alzheimer's should be under a doctor's care. He or she may see a primary care doctor or a specialist, such as a neurologist, geriatric psychiatrist, or geriatrician. The doctor can treat the person's physical and behavioral problems, answer questions, and refer the patient and caregiver to other sources of help.

Medications for Alzheimer's

Currently, no treatment can stop Alzheimer's disease. However, four medications are used to treat its symptoms. These medicines may help maintain thinking, memory, and speaking skills for a limited time. They work by regulating certain chemicals in the brain. Most of these medicines work best for people in the early or middle stages of the disease.

For people with mild to moderate Alzheimer's, donepezil (Aricept®), rivastigmine (Exelon®), or galantamine (Razadyne®) may help. Donepezil is also approved to treat symptoms of moderate to severe Alzheimer's. Another drug, memantine (Namenda®), is used to treat symptoms of moderate to severe Alzheimer's, although it also has limited effects.

All of these medicines have possible side effects, including nausea, vomiting, diarrhea, and loss of appetite. You should report any unusual symptoms to a doctor right away. It is important to follow a doctor's instructions when taking any medication.

Scientists are testing many new drugs and other treatments to see if they can help slow, delay, or prevent Alzheimer's disease.

Managing Behavioral Symptoms

Certain medicines and other approaches can help control the behavioral symptoms of Alzheimer's disease. These symptoms include sleeplessness, agitation, wandering, anxiety, anger, and depression. Treating these symptoms often makes people with Alzheimer's disease more comfortable and makes their care easier for caregivers.

Memory Aids

Memory aids may help some people who have mild Alzheimer's disease with day-to-day living. A calendar, list of daily plans, notes about simple safety measures, and written directions describing how to use common household items can be useful.

Help for Caregivers

Caring for a person with Alzheimer's can have high physical, emotional, and financial costs. The demands of day-to-day care, changing family roles, and difficult decisions about placement in a care facility can be hard to handle.

Sometimes, taking care of the person with Alzheimer's makes caregivers feel good because they are providing love and comfort. At other times, it can be overwhelming. Changes in the person can be hard to understand and cope with.

Here are some ways for caregivers of people with Alzheimer's to get help.

- Ask family and friends to help out in specific ways, like making a meal or visiting the person while they take a break.
- Join a caregivers' support group.
- Use home health care, adult day care, and respite services.

Chapter 6: Research

Thirty years ago, we knew very little about Alzheimer's disease. Since then, scientists have made important advances. Research supported by the National Institutes of Health (NIH) and other organizations has expanded knowledge of brain function in healthy older people, identified ways that may lessen age-related cognitive decline, and deepened our understanding of Alzheimer's.

Many scientists and physicians are working together to untangle the genetic, biological, and environmental factors that might cause Alzheimer's disease. This effort is bringing us closer to better managing and, ultimately, preventing this devastating disease.

Types of Research

Different types of research—basic, translational, and clinical research—are conducted to find ways to treat, delay, or prevent Alzheimer's disease.

- Basic research helps scientists gain new knowledge about a disease process, including how and why it starts and progresses.

- <u>Translational research</u> grows out of basic research. It creates new medicines, devices, or behavioral interventions aimed at preventing, diagnosing, or treating a disease.
- <u>Clinical research</u> is medical research involving people. It includes clinical studies, which observe and gather information about large groups of people. It also includes clinical trials, which test a medicine, therapy, medical device, or behavior in people to see if it is safe and effective.

Basic Research

Basic research seeks to identify the cellular, molecular, and genetic processes that lead to Alzheimer's disease. Basic research has focused on two of the main signs of Alzheimer's disease in the brain: plaques and tangles. Plaques are made of a protein called beta-amyloid and form abnormal clumps among cells of the brain. Tangles are made from a protein called tau and form twisted bundles of fibers within nerve cells in the brain.

Scientists are studying the ways in which plaques and tangles damage nerve cells in the brain. They can now see beta-amyloid plaques by making images of the brains of living people. Such imaging has led to clinical trials that are looking at ways to remove beta-amyloid from the human brain or halt its production before more brain damage occurs.

Scientists are also exploring the very earliest brain changes in the disease process. Findings will help them better understand the causes of Alzheimer's. As they learn more, they are likely to come up with better targets for further research. Over time, this might lead to more effective therapies to delay or prevent the disease.

Genetics is another important area of basic research. Discovering more about the role of Alzheimer's risk-factor genes will help researchers answers questions such as "What makes the disease process begin?" and "Why do some people with memory and other thinking problems develop Alzheimer's disease while others do not?"

Genetics research helps scientists learn how risk-factor genes interact with other genes and lifestyle or environmental factors to affect Alzheimer's risk. This research also helps scientists identify people who are at high risk for developing Alzheimer's and focus on new prevention and treatment approaches.

Translational Research

Translational research allows new knowledge from basic research to be applied to a clinical research setting. An important goal of Alzheimer's translational research is to increase the number and variety of potential new medicines and other interventions that are approved for testing in humans. Scientists also examine medicines approved to treat other diseases to see they might be effective in people with Alzheimer's.

The most promising interventions are tested in test-tube and animal studies to make sure they are safe and effective. Currently, a number of different substances are under development that may one day be used to treat the symptoms of Alzheimer's disease or mild cognitive impairment (MCI).

Clinical Research

Clinical research is medical research involving people. It includes clinical studies, which observe and gather information about large groups of people. It also includes clinical trials, which test medicines, therapies, medical devices, or behaviors in people to see if they are safe and effective.

Clinical trials are the best way to find out whether a particular intervention actually slows, delays, or prevents Alzheimer's disease. Trials may compare a potential new treatment with a standard treatment or placebo (mock treatment). Or, they may study whether a certain behavior or condition affects the progress of Alzheimer's or the chances of developing it.

NIH, drug companies, and other research organizations are conducting many clinical trials to test possible new treatments that may

- improve memory, thinking, and reasoning skills in people with Alzheimer's or mild cognitive impairment
- relieve the behavior problems of Alzheimer's, such as aggression and agitation
- delay the progression from mild cognitive impairment (MCI) to Alzheimer's
- prevent Alzheimer's disease.

A wide variety of interventions are being tested in clinical trials. They include experimental drugs as well as non-drug approaches. New medicines being tested include

- intravenous Immunoglobulin (IVIg), a blood product administered intravenously.

It contains naturally occurring antibodies against beta-amyloid.
- resveratrol, a dietary supplement that contains a compound found in red grapes and red wine. It may help protect the brain.
- a nasal-spray form of the hormone insulin. It might delay memory loss and preserve general cognition.

Chapter 7: Participating in Research

People with Alzheimer's disease, those with MCI, those with a family history of Alzheimer's, and healthy people with no memory problems who want to help scientists test new treatments may be able to take part in clinical trials. Participants in clinical trials help scientists learn about the brain in healthy aging as well as what happens in Alzheimer's. Results of these trials are used to improve prevention and treatment methods.

The Alzheimer's Disease Education and Referral (ADEAR) Center's clinical trials finder makes it easy for people to find out about studies that are sponsored by the federal government and private companies. It includes studies testing new ways to detect, treat, delay, and prevent Alzheimer's disease, other dementias, and MCI.

To find out more about Alzheimer's clinical trials, talk to your health care provider or contact the ADEAR Center at 1-800-438-4380.

Chapter 8: Additional Resources

The Alzheimer's Disease Education and Referral (ADEAR) Center is a service of the National Institute on Aging (NIA), one of the Federal Government's National Institutes of Health and part of the U.S. Department of Health and Human Services. The NIA conducts and supports research about health issues for older people and is the primary Federal agency for Alzheimer's disease research.

Visit the ADEAR Center website to find current, comprehensive, unbiased information about Alzheimer's disease. All our information and materials about the search for causes, treatment, cures, and better diagnostic tools are carefully researched and thoroughly reviewed by NIA scientists and health communicators for accuracy and integrity.

You can also call 1-800-438-4380 to talk to ADEAR Center Information Specialists to assist you with

- answers to your specific questions about Alzheimer's disease
- free publications about Alzheimer's symptoms, diagnosis, related disorders, risk factors, treatment, caregiving tips, home safety tips, and research

- referrals to local supportive services and Alzheimer's Disease Centers that specialize in research and diagnosis
- clinical trials information
- training materials, guidelines, and news updates
- Spanish language resources

To contact the ADEAR Center, call 1-800-438-4380 (toll-free) or go to www.nia.nih.gov/alzheimers.

Chapter 9: Frequently Asked Questions

1. What is Alzheimer's disease?

Alzheimer's disease is a brain disease that slowly destroys memory and thinking skills and, eventually, the ability to carry out the simplest tasks. It begins slowly and gets worse over time. Currently, it has no cure. Alzheimer's disease is the most common cause of dementia in older people.

2. What is dementia?

Dementia is a loss of thinking, remembering, and reasoning skills that interferes with a person's daily life and activities. Alzheimer's disease is the most common cause of dementia among older people. Dementia ranges in severity from the mild stage, when it is just beginning to affect a person's functioning, to the severe stage, when the person must depend completely on others for care.

3. How many people in the United States have Alzheimer's disease?

Estimates vary, but experts suggest that as many as 5.1 million people in the United States may have Alzheimer's disease.

4. What is mild cognitive impairment?

Mild cognitive impairment, or MCI, is a condition that can be an early sign of Alzheimer's disease—but not everyone with MCI will develop Alzheimer's. People with MCI can still take care of themselves and do their normal activities. Signs of MCI may include

- losing things often
- forgetting to go to events and appointments
- having more trouble coming up with words than other people the same age.

5. What is typically the first sign of Alzheimer's disease?

Memory problems are typically one of the first signs of Alzheimer's disease. A person in the early (mild) stage of Alzheimer's disease may

- find it hard to remember things
- ask the same questions over and over

- get lost
- lose things or put them in odd places
- have trouble handling money and paying bills
- take longer than normal to finish daily tasks.

Other thinking problems besides memory loss may be the first sign of Alzheimer's disease. A person may have trouble finding the right words, vision and spatial issues, or impaired reasoning or judgment. He or she may also have some mood or personality changes.

6. What are the stages in the development of Alzheimer's disease?

Alzheimer's disease has three stages: early (also called mild), middle (moderate), and late (severe).

A person in the early stage of Alzheimer's may
- find it hard to remember things
- ask the same questions over and over
- lose things
- have trouble handling money and paying bills.

As Alzheimer's disease progresses to the middle stage, memory loss and confusion grow worse, and people may have problems recognizing family and friends. Other symptoms are this stage include

- diffculty learning new things and coping with new situations
- trouble carrying out tasks that involve multiple steps, like getting dressed
- forgetting the names of common things
- wandering away from home.

As Alzheimer's disease becomes more severe, people lose the ability to communicate. They may sleep more, lose weight, and have trouble swallowing. Often they are incontinent—they cannot control their bladder and/or bowels. Eventually, they need total care.

7. What changes in the brain happen to people with Alzheimer's disease?

Although we still don't know how Alzheimer's disease begins, it seems likely that damage to the brain starts 10 years or more before problems become obvious. During the earliest stage of Alzheimer's, people are free of symptoms, but harmful changes are taking place in the brain. Abnormal protein deposits form amyloid plaques and neurofibrillary tangles in the brain. Once-healthy nerve cells lose their ability to function and communicate with each other, and eventually they die.

As nerve cells in the brain die, parts of the brain begin to shrink. By the final stage of Alzheimer's, damage is widespread, and brain tissue has shrunk significantly.

8. What causes Alzheimer's disease?

Scientists do not yet fully understand what causes Alzheimer's disease. It is likely that the causes include some mix of genetic, environmental, and lifestyle factors. These factors affect each person differently.

Increasing age is the most important known risk factor for Alzheimer's disease. Lifestyle factors, such as diet and physical exercise, and long-term health conditions, like high blood pressure and diabetes, might also play a role in the risk of developing Alzheimer's disease.

9. If a family member has Alzheimer's disease, will I get it, too?

Just because a family member has Alzheimer's disease does not mean that you will get it, too. A rare form of Alzheimer's disease, called early-onset familial Alzheimer's, is inherited. It occurs in people between the ages of 30 and 60 and is caused by mutations, or changes, in certain genes.

Most cases of Alzheimer's are late-onset. They occur after age 60 and usually have no obvious family pattern. However, genetic factors appear to increase a person's risk of developing late-onset Alzheimer's.

10. If you become forgetful as you get older, does that mean you will get Alzheimer's disease?

Not all memory problems are caused by Alzheimer's disease. Mild forgetfulness can be a normal part of aging. Sometimes memory problems are related to health issues that are treatable. For example, medication side effects, vitamin B12 deficiency, or liver or kidney disorders can lead to memory loss or possibly dementia. Emotional problems, such as stress, anxiety, or depression, can also make a person more forgetful and may be mistaken for dementia.

If you or someone in your family thinks your forgetfulness is getting in the way of your normal routine, it's time to see your doctor. He or she can find out what's causing these problems.

11. How is Alzheimer's disease diagnosed?

The only definitive way to diagnose Alzheimer's disease is to find out whether plaques and tangles exist in brain tissue. To look at brain tissue, doctors perform a brain autopsy, an examination of the brain done after a person dies. To diagnose Alzheimer's disease, doctors may

- ask questions about overall health, past medical problems, ability to carry out daily activities, and changes in behavior and personality
- conduct tests to measure memory, problem solving, attention, counting, and language skills
- carry out standard medical tests, such as blood and urine tests
- perform brain scans to look for anything in the brain that does not look normal.

12. Why is early diagnosis of Alzheimer's important?

An early, accurate diagnosis of Alzheimer's disease helps people and their families plan for the future. It gives them time to discuss care options, find support, and make legal and financial arrangements while the person with Alzheimer's can still take part in making decisions. Also, even though no medicine or other treatment can stop or slow the disease, early diagnosis offers the best chance to treat the symptoms.

13. How long do people live after getting diagnosed with Alzheimer's?

The time from diagnosis of Alzheimer's disease to death varies. It can be as little as 3 or 4 years if the person is over 80 years old when diagnosed or as long as 10 years or more if the person is younger.

14. Are there any medicines to treat Alzheimer's disease?

Currently, no treatment can stop Alzheimer's disease. However, four medications are used to treat its symptoms. These medicines may help maintain thinking, memory, and speaking skills for a limited time. They work by regulating certain chemicals in the brain. Most of these medicines work best for people in the early or middle stages of the disease.

For people with mild or moderate Alzheimer's, donepezil (Aricept®), rivastigmine (Exelon®), or galantamine (Razadyne®) may help. Donepezil is also approved to treat symptoms of moderate to severe Alzheimer's. Another drug, memantine (Namenda®), is used to treat symptoms of moderate to severe Alzheimer's, although it also has limited effects. All of these medicines have possible side effects.

Certain medicines and other approaches can help control the behavioral symptoms of Alzheimer's disease. These symptoms include sleeplessness, agitation, wandering, anxiety, anger, and depression.

15. Is there anything I can do to prevent Alzheimer's disease?

Currently, no medicines or treatments are known to prevent Alzheimer's disease, but scientists are studying many possibilities. These possibilities include lifestyle factors such as exercise and physical activity, a healthy diet, and mentally stimulating activities.

In addition to lifestyle factors, scientists have found clues that some long-term health conditions, like heart disease, high blood pressure, and diabetes, are related to Alzheimer's disease. It's possible that controlling these conditions will reduce the risk of developing Alzheimer's.

16. Can exercising prevent Alzheimer's disease?

Research suggests that exercise may play a role in reducing risk for Alzheimer's disease. Animal studies show that exercise increases both the number of small blood vessels that supply blood to the brain and the number of connections between nerve cells in older rats and mice. In addition, researchers have found that exercise raises the level of a nerve growth factor (a protein key to brain health) in an area of the brain that is important to memory and learning. Researchers have also shown that exercise can stimulate the human brain's ability to maintain old network connections and make new ones.

17. Can controlling certain diseases protect against Alzheimer's?

Age-related diseases and conditions—such as vascular disease, high blood pressure, heart disease, and diabetes—may increase the risk of Alzheimer's. Many studies are looking at whether this risk can be reduced by preventing or controlling these diseases and conditions.

For example, one clinical trial is looking at how lowering blood pressure to or below current recommended levels may affect cognitive decline and the development of MCI (mild cognitive impairment) and Alzheimer's disease. Participants are older adults with high systolic (upper number) blood pressure who have a history of heart disease or stroke, or are at risk for those conditions.

Diabetes is another disease that has been linked to Alzheimer's. Past research suggests that abnormal insulin production contributes to Alzheimer's-related brain changes.

(Insulin is the hormone involved in diabetes.) Diabetes treatments have been tested in people with Alzheimer's, but the results have not been conclusive.

18. Can eating certain foods prevent Alzheimer's disease?

A number of studies suggest that eating certain foods may help keep the brain healthy—and that others can be harmful. Researchers are looking at whether a healthy diet—one that includes lots of fruits, vegetables, and whole grains and is low in fat and added sugar—can help prevent Alzheimer's.

19. Can you prevent Alzheimer's by keeping your brain active?

Keeping the mind sharp—through social engagement or intellectual stimulation—is associated with a lower risk of Alzheimer's disease. Activities like working, volunteering, reading, going to lectures, and playing computer and other games are being studied to see if they might help prevent Alzheimer's. But we do not know with certainty whether these activities can actually prevent Alzheimer's.

20. What is basic research and why is it an important part of Alzheimer's disease research?

Basic research helps scientists gain new knowledge about a disease process, including how and why it starts and progresses. In Alzheimer's disease, basic search seeks to identify the cellular, molecular, and genetic processes that lead to the disease. For example, scientists are studying

- the ways in which plaques and tangles damage nerve cells in the brain
- the very earliest brain changes in the disease process
- the role of Alzheimer's risk-factor genes in the development of the disease
- how risk-factor genes interact with other genes and lifestyle or environmental factors to affect Alzheimer's risk.

21. What is translational research and why is it an important part of Alzheimer's disease research?

Translational research grows out of basic research. It creates new medicines, devices, or behavioral interventions aimed at preventing, diagnosing, or treating a disease. An important goal of Alzheimer's translational research is to increase the number and variety of potential new medicines and other interventions that are approved for testing in humans. Scientists also examine medicines approved to treat other diseases to see they might be effective in people with Alzheimer's.

The most promising interventions are tested in test-tube and animal studies to make sure they are safe and effective. Currently, a number of different substances are under development that may one day be used to treat the symptoms of Alzheimer's disease or mild cognitive impairment.

22. What is clinical research and why is it an important part of Alzheimer's disease research?

Clinical research is medical research involving people. It includes clinical studies, which observe and gather information about large groups of people. It also includes clinical trials, which test a medicine, therapy, medical device, or behavior in people to see if it is safe and effective.

Clinical trials are the best way to find out whether a particular intervention actually slows, delays, or prevents Alzheimer's disease. Trials may compare a potential new treatment with a standard treatment or placebo (mock treatment). Or, they may study whether a certain behavior or condition affects the progress of Alzheimer's or the chances of developing it.

23. How can people help test possible new treatments for Alzheimer's?

People with Alzheimer's disease, those with mild cognitive impairment, those with a family history of Alzheimer's, and healthy people with no memory problems who want to help scientists test new treatments may be able to take part in clinical trials. Participants in clinical trials help scientists learn about the brain in healthy aging as well as what happens in Alzheimer's. Results of these trials are used to improve prevention and treatment methods.

To find out more about Alzheimer's clinical trials, talk to your health care provider or contact the <u>Alzheimer's Disease Education and Referral (ADEAR) Center</u> at 1-800-438-4380.

Other MedicalCenter.com Publications

The Key Facts on Arthritis

The Key Facts on Breast Cancer

The Key Facts on Medicare

All Titles Can Be Found at

www.Amazon.com

www.MedicalCenter.com